Contents

PREFACE

The decision to write this handbook came after 20 years of healthcare experience, both in physician offices, hospitals and senior long term care settings.

In that time, I personally witnessed a lot of sad situations happen to a variety of different families and patients. I could see the struggle that families went through to make the best decisions for their loved ones, in spite of so much confusing direction.

My hope is that this handbook can help them successfully navigate our healthcare system.

After dealing with a variety of patients, physicians, hospital social workers, and insurance companies with success, I decided to use my knowledge to help more people and their families have the needed information to understand our very complex healthcare system.

Daily I've witnessed the confusion that families go through while trying to make the best medical decision for their loved ones. I've seen the agony and frustration they experience in trying to get accurate information.

Since healthcare in America has become a very complex maze, and is a <u>BUSINESS</u>, it can be very hard to navigate.

Furthermore, as each healthcare entity has a different financial agenda, with the common goal being to make a profit, you must know what the agenda is to ensure that you are truly making decisions that benefit your loved one, and not simply promoting someone's bottom line.

I dedicate this book to everyone attempting to navigate our healthcare system in America, as well as the kindhearted, ethical, and caring medical professionals that want to provide the best possible health care for their patients.

They are truly angels walking among us!

INTRODUCTION

Aging in America may seem confusing to many seniors and the members of their support systems. Why can't they get a straight answer?

Simply put, it is because our healthcare system in America is a business and all businesses are trying to make a profit.

Therefore, many of the medical professionals and entities we trust have a financial agenda. Numbers not patients, bring profits. So when you know that you are a number, you can better understand why you are being directed in a specific direction.

I've seen seniors and their families go through extreme anxiety due to the choices offered to them by their physicians, hospitals, and insurance companies.

Many times these families do not even know they have other alternatives than the options they are being given. Therefore, many people suffer physical and financial consequences that could have been avoided.

Unfortunately, seniors who have no one to protect them suffer even greater injustices. I could give countless examples that have broken my heart over the years, but instead would prefer to give inside information on how to avoid the agendas of providers that could actually unintentionally or intentionally cause harm to you or your loved one.

If you know why you're being directed in one place over another, or understand why you're not being given some choices at all, hopefully it can help to make better decisions for you or your loved one. Many times I hear the same question from patients and their families:

Why did one provider only give me certain options?

Why did one provider make one recommendation and another one a completely different one?

This handbook is intended to help you make the best possible healthcare decisions for you or your aging loved one.

DISCLAIMER

AGING IN AMERICA

WHAT *YOU NEED TO KNOW* ABOUT NAVIGATING OUR HEALTHCARE SYSTEM

A *PRACTICAL GUIDE* TO HELP FAMILIES MAKE THE BEST CHOICES FOR THEIR AGING LOVED ONES

The author of this book does not dispense medical advice nor prescribe the use of any technique as a form of treatment for physical, emotional, or medical problems without the advice of a physician, either directly or indirectly.

The author does not give legal advice regarding Medicare or Medicaid and / or in the selecting of any specific insurance entity. Any state or federally mandated programs must be verified with the local state or federal government representatives.

The author's intent is to offer information on the healthcare industry in a practical and useful way. The referrals to experts still require personal research in deciding the best tools and resources to select for any individual situation.

The author assumes no personal or financial liability for any choices that may be decided upon after reading this information.

AGING IN AMERICA

WHAT YOU *NEED TO KNOW* ABOUT NAVIGATING
OUR HEALTHCARE SYSTEM

CHAPTER 1

CHOOSING THE BEST PRIMARY CARE PHYSICIAN

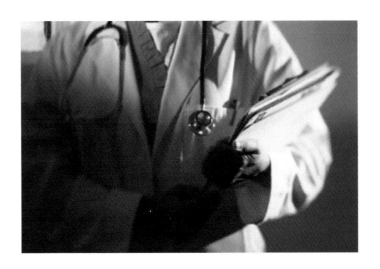

*Learn how to select the best physician for
your health care journey.*

CHOOSING A PRIMARY CARE PHYSICIAN

Why start with choosing a primary care physician?

Simply put, a primary care physician is the co-pilot of every person's healthcare journey.

Many seniors choose a physician, or are assigned one by an insurance company, when relatively healthy, or for a temporary medical condition.

The physician may have been recommended by a friend, or have been assigned by the insurance company, and many have not evaluated the doctor to make sure they have the best one.

For many seniors their doctor can become a part of their entire life, and very much like a member of the family, and by the time the senior is now aging, their primary physician is also.

Many older physicians do *NOT* still have active hospital privileges and some are not always up to date with the newest and best practices in medicine. Why is this so important?

Once a senior has developed certain chronic medical conditions, such as high blood pressure, diabetes, chronic heart failure that require prescription management, this is where a physician that hasn't kept up with the latest information may be recommending outdated drugs or treatments, and may not be aware of the most current medication interactions and procedures.

Most often, the senior may have a loyalty to their physician, even if they aren't feeling better, due to

the span of history they share. However, in the case of a medical emergency requiring a hospital or rehabilitation stay, this loyalty towards their doctor will not serve them well.

Unless a person has a lot of health issues, most only see their primary care physician a few times of year at best, and for a few brief minutes, at best.

In the event of a sudden medical emergency or accident, the primary care physician becomes the MOST important person on the medical team. Therefore, choosing a primary physician that is not only competent and well trained can drastically affect the future choices and options a person will have available.

Since most humans are instilled with instincts that we will all live forever and never get ill, we usually don't think about the doctor we've chosen until we need them.

Your primary care physician, who is the ultimate manager of your health journey, is the one that will be helping you decide what medications are needed, and in the event of a hospital stay will be the key person directing you or a loved one's recovery.

A primary care physician can become a friend, concerned for your overall wellness, however SHOULD also be someone you can rely upon in the event of an unforeseen major illness, or medical emergency.

This choice is so crucial because it's important that the physician you've chosen is in agreement with your wishes.

Some have found out only after they get taken to the hospital that their doctor does not have hospital privileges at all, or may not even be allowed at the hospital of their choice. Then they are even more surprised to find out that their care decisions are now being assigned to a virtual stranger.

So if a senior is attached to a physician that does NOT have hospital privileges, what can be done? It's recommended keeping the older doctor as a friend, invite them over for the holidays if you like, however, find and add a Board Certified Physician that can manage the seniors changing medical needs more competently and up to date.

Furthermore, most primary care physicians have alliances they make with specific hospitals, hospitalist physicians, rehabilitation centers, home health agencies, and Medicare and Medicaid replacement Insurance companies. Why do they form these alliances?

Most physicians choose to align themselves with quality care organizations to protect them from malpractice claims and a damaging reputation.

However, for some physicians, the shrinking pay and rising operational expenses make them make some decisions based on the money their alliances will pay them.

Due to the challenges of making money as a physician, many doctors have changed their practices to only treat patients on an outpatient basis, in their offices, while others have decided on only having a hospital based practice. Some doctors have chosen a hybrid method, in which they treat their patients in an outpatient setting but also follow them to the local hospitals and rehabilitation centers.

Across the nation, physicians are dealing with shrinking reimbursements from most insurance companies, higher malpractice insurance costs and the daily challenges of running an office with ever increasing overhead.

Also, the physicians who DO take care of their patients while in a Hospital and/or Skilled Nursing and Rehab Centers like to have most of their patients in a convenient area, to maximize their very limited time.

Therefore, due to the shrinking income they're struggling with, these alliances pay their physicians as a medical director a monthly stipend or bonus, which can benefit as extra income for their practice. This may be a key factor as to WHY a physician is making a referral to a certain home care agency, hospital or rehabilitation center.

Usually a medical directorship or advisory position can pay a physician from $500.00 to $15000.00 per month, per entity (Hospital, Skilled Nursing Center, Home Health Agency, etc) depending on the area in the country. Therefore, on a yearly basis this income collectively becomes a huge asset.

Contrary to what most people may stereotypically assume, not all physicians are rich, and some have enormous debt loads. Therefore, these additional incomes are something that they vehemently protect. For instance, if a rehab center is looking at hiring a different Medical Director, to preserve this income, they will be more feverishly looking for one of their patients to admit there, to reaffirm their worth, and preserve their job and income with that rehab center.

Also, some physicians have become contracted providers with Medicare and Medicaid Advantage Plans (HMO's), and receive money for their patient office visits, as well as a monthly amount per patient they have with said HMO Insurance Company. This payment per patient payment can range from $5.00 to $30.00 or more, per patient per month, which is commonly known as a monthly capped amount. They receive this monthly patient capped income from the Insurance companies, regardless if they've seen any of these patients that are members of the insurance company during the month, or not.

These Insurance Companies, who accept federal Medicare money and state Medicaid money are trying to maximize their profits, i.e. make their business profitable. Therefore, they require certain services and specialties to be authorized, and impose limitations on the physicians as to what they are allowed to offer their patients, *and in some cases, despite what a patient's medical condition requires.*

Thus, many physicians struggle as they try to manage their patient's wellness within the limitations imposed upon them by the various Insurance companies. At times this develops into situations where they are not able to practice medicine in the way that they've been trained and know to be more accurate.

For example, some Insurance contracts penalize a physician financially when they order certain costly tests, specialist consultations, rehab or home health services, and/or simply deny authorization for some or all of these services.

At times, when a physician wants their patients to have medical assistance in the home, an expensive medication, a specialty test or some other service or procedure that can make a difference in their health, they are simply not allowed to order these services.

What is maddening is that many of these services are entitlements allowed under straight Medicare or Medicaid. Our government agencies actually give an incentive to these insurance companies to manage the distribution of benefits to the recipients entitled, but sadly, many find very legal and ingenious ways to avoid authorizing what they are required to do. With minimal oversight from the government, the Insurance companies have been able to get away with NOT providing members what their physician feels they need.

Many times a physician's referrals can have financial consequences for them, and can influence the referrals they make. All physicians take an oath to "cause no harm," however, may struggle with their oath and the reality of making a profitable living at the same time.

Simply put, physicians are running a *BUSINESS* as well.

Therefore, the options that will be offered a patient while in the community or in the event of a hospital stay are always directed by the primary care physician, as long as they have *ACTIVE* hospital privileges.

If a primary care physician does <u>NOT</u> have hospital privileges, then a hospitalist physician will assume this role during the hospital stay. This virtual stranger will now be calling all the shots during the entire hospital stay, without having a previous understanding of the patient's medical history.

Hospitalist physicians can be either an independent physician that accepts patients whose physicians don't round in hospitals, or be employed by the hospital primarily and do not have any community offices.

While in the hospital, a primary care physician or hospitalist physician will be making medical decisions such as what tests, medications, specialty consultations, are needed.

This is where the alliances come into the picture. If the physician taking care of a patient in the hospital is the Medical Director of a certain skilled nursing center, they usually try to direct to those centers they work with. HOPEFULLY, it's one preferred and is convenient to your support system.

Similarly, they usually follow suit if the patient is being discharged home, and will write an order for the company they work with, or is paying them a monthly stipend.

If there is a Commercial Insurance, Medicare or Medicaid replacement HMO, the options become even more limited. The influence of Medicare

Advantage Plans will be covered in subsequent chapters.

Since a primary care physician is so crucial to anyone's future wellness, how can the best one be chosen?

There are many ways to obtain the best recommendations. Word of mouth is always an excellent way, however, the best recommendations come from someone who works in healthcare. Many healthcare employees have learned which physicians are the most ethical, and which may be best suited for someone's personal preferences (man, woman, nationality, etc) and Insurance company.

Many have learned from some of their neighbors and friends experiences which ones are of a higher expertise and integrity. Most hospitals, senior centers and assisted living communities sometimes offer lectures and an opportunity to meet the physicians personally. At these sessions a potential patient has the opportunity to know that physician, and ask questions without having to set an appointment in their office.

With the influence of the internet, there are many different internet sites that grade and judge the quality of all local physicians, and include any pending malpractice claims against them.

This decision is so important to anyone's future health choices that a checklist is included to best judge weather a physician would be the best for you or a loved one, and be willing to work in harmony with your wishes.

Because you usually only have a very short time during an appointment to discuss specifics with any physician, a lot of the needed information can be gathered by looking around the office or asking the staff.

Additionally, most local hospitals have websites that list the physicians that have privileges with them, including their specialties, training, and usually a picture.

USEFUL TIPS

1. Do your research. Investigate a doctor you may be interested in online, and through word of mouth BEFORE you set an appointment. Ask if they are board certified and in what specialties (Board Certified physicians have additional training and testing).

2. <u>INTERVIEW THE PHYSICIAN (see Physician Interview form)</u> Find out what Hospitals, Nursing centers and Home Health agencies they primarily work with.

3. Do your research on the hospital and Rehab & nursing centers, and home health agencies online. Every state has an organization that survey these centers and agencies to judge what, if any, deficiencies they have.

4. Visit the hospitals and skilled nursing centers that THIS PHYSICIAN is primarily affiliated with.

5. Look very carefully at the brochures that are in your Drs. waiting room, as this is a clue to observe if your doctor has a few alliances, or "plays the Medical Director game" with many companies. This may become important as it may affect referrals to affiliates later on when needed.

6. It's also critical to know how many Medicare and Medicaid HMO's they are promoting, which again will limit your choices in the event of an emergency.

7. If the physician is owned by any Medicare Advantage Plan Insurance Companies, they may have an Insurance case manager that all authorizations go through.

8. It's also good to know if the physician practice is owned by any Hospitals. Hospitals have been purchasing some physician offices as well, and hopefully it is a hospital that you like, as you will be directed there, and to any other services they offer.

__Make sure to bring a current medication listing including vitamin supplements that are being taken to save the physician time.__

__Also, write down any specific questions about your health you may have for the physician in advance.__

When a physician is owned by an Insurance company, sometimes, they are not at liberty at times to order certain tests or services their patients need as the insurance company must require prior approval.

When a Hospital owns a Dr.'s practice, the physician is not usually at liberty to make recommendations to any Hospital, Skilled Nursing center, or ancillary service other than the ones the Hospital owns.

There have been many cases where a physician, especially the ones owned by an Insurance company, may try to convince a patient that they don't need what the rest of the healthcare providers are saying they do.

For example, a physician once told a 66 year old woman that had just had a hip surgery that she didn't require physical therapy at a rehab center because she smoked and instead should just call in Hospice. Thankfully, the family was educated about their rights and the physician was forced to order and authorize the services she needed. Her Medicare Advantage Plan's Case Manager was not happy. The Physician went so far as to complain to my Administrator at the time about me informing the family of their rights.

Sadly, these cases are not isolated and many seniors and families have found out while in the midst of a crisis that their physician was not the best choice for them.

If you don't feel comfortable with your primary care physician for any reason you should continue your search. What is chiefly important is that whomever is chosen will have your best interests at heart and not their own pocketbook.

If your Medicare Advantage Plan has assigned a doctor that makes you uncomfortable for any reason, call the customer service line immediately, as they can usually offer to assign another doctor.

PHYSICIAN INTERVIEW FORM

(LOOK AROUND THE OFFICE FOR ANSWERS)

What is the average age of his/her patient practice?

_____

What Hospital (s) do they admit to mostly? If they don't have hospital privileges, which Dr. (s) do they refer to, and what hospital do they work out of?

_____

What Skilled Nursing & Rehab Centers / "Nursing Homes" do they refer to? _____

Are they Medical Director / Advisor of any of them?

_____

What Home Health Agencies does he/she work with, and are they Director of any? _____

Is he/she Board Certified? _____
Any specialty training? _____

Are they open to natural and alternative methods of treatments? _____

Are they part of any Medicare / Medicaid Advantage Plans / HMO? _____

Are the majority of their patients on Original Medicare or Medicare Advantage Plans?

Many have found out the hard way that the hospital, skilled nursing centers, and home care agencies their primary care physician has referred them to, is substandard. Selecting the best partner for your healthcare journey can be done by researching physicians and their affiliations CAREFULLY.

For example, if a Dr. does a lot of clinical drug trials, which they get paid for by the pharmaceutical companies, may be prescribing more medications than needed. Also, some physicians, especially the ones that are NOT board certified have been known to overmedicate their patients, and/or prescribe outdated medications, which can lead to many unpleasant complications and side effects.

In one case, if a primary care physician who is the Medical director of a respiratory hospital, has consistently directed patients there, even if it may NOT be medically necessary, and especially when the census or patient occupancy is low.

In addition, there are certain times of the year when hospitals and skilled nursing centers have more open beds. This is the time when you or a loved one may be directed to a certain place, even if it's not medically necessary, or the recovery care could be handled at home.

In another case, a nursing home resident whose family lived out of town and went to the hospital to be treated for pneumonia. Because the census (occupancy rate) was low at his primary care physician's respiratory hospital affiliate which he was the medical director of, the patient was sent to that hospital, even though he did not meet the criteria, and his needs could easily be met at his nursing home, which had become his long term home.

Another example of how a physician can control what type of care you receive is evidenced by one physician whose husband is a Gastroenterologist and almost all of this doctor's nursing home residents get a standard order for a GI consult, by her husband, when they are admitted to the hospital. This is to see if they need a feeding tube in their stomach, whether they can swallow or not. A feeding tube, or peg tube are generally used to feed a patient when they cannot swallow any longer on their own. It is known by the hospital staff that this physician is helping her husband pay for their lifestyle by the choice of her recommendations for her nursing home patients, EVERY ONE.

In one case, her patient passed EVERY swallow test, and this physician was still insisting that the patient receive a feeding tube. Luckily, the hospital staff and family intervened so that this sweet senior who loved her sweets would not lose access to them.

There are seasonal changes that can affect how a physician directs their patients as well. For some areas, the slow season in some places may be during the summer, which means the physicians are under more pressure than usual from their affiliates to send them business, or patients. Thus, if you observe that the hospital you or your loved one is in seems highly quiet, it could be that they are having a slow time of the year for them. Be even more vigilant that the direction you or your loved one is sent are in direct harmony with your wishes.

As previously discussed, when a physician is the Medical Director of a Rehab center, these entities sometimes pay them thousands of dollars monthly, and expect the doctor to keep them busy with their patients. So during the slow times of the year, these doctors are under even more pressure to deliver patients to them, and that could end up being you or your loved one, despite your objections.

** <u>If you ever find yourself in this situation, feel free to ask to speak with a social worker or case manager that works for the hospital, as they can become an advocate for you or your loved one's behalf.</u> **

Board Certified physicians are especially careful to align themselves with the providers known for giving the highest quality of care and with better reviews from the state agencies. They not only have their medical license and board status to protect, but also run the risk of more malpractice claims when choosing providers to align their practice with.

Older physicians that a senior may have had for many years, and loves, may not be the best choice to manage them in a hospital setting, if that becomes necessary. Therefore, the best recommendation for a high quality ethical physician is one that is Board Certified, has a lower percentage of Managed Care Insurance companies that they contract with, and is trained at handling patients during a hospital stay, or has Board Certified hospitalists that they refer to.

With some research, and careful conversation, you can be certain that your medical care is in the best of hands if a hospital stay or more complex medical care is necessary.

Some websites below can give a physician's info:

www.healthgrades.com

www.ratemds.com

www.vitals.com

www.informedpatient.org

www.hca.com

www.baycare.org

www.va.gov

AGING IN AMERICA

WHAT YOU *NEED TO KNOW* ABOUT NAVIGATING OUR HEALTHCARE SYSTEM

CHAPTER 2

TOUR INDEPENDENT, ASSISTED & SKILLED NURSING/REHAB CENTERS *BEFORE NEEDED*

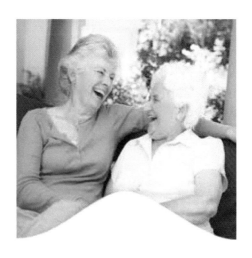

Tips for choosing the right long term care housing!

.

Fact: Some Seniors live 3-5 years longer when living in a long term care setting.

Although most seniors as they are aging are convinced that they will retire and die at home, and may say, "I'm only leaving my home feet first". This is simply a denial of the mind, as most people do not have this experience in their golden years.

Many people do not want to be reminded that they are aging, and simply avoid doing any preventative research that can have a huge impact on their future lives. Some very practical seniors have decided voluntarily to make their preparations on their own. To them ~ I say – Bravo!

The statistics show that 70 % of Americans will require help with the activities of daily living (ADL's) at some future point in time. There are six basic ADLs: eating, bathing, dressing, toileting, transferring (walking) and continence.

When a family accepts that their loved one will need additional help at some future point in the future, most likely in a healthcare center, it becomes reasonable to begin touring centers to be in a position to choose the best one.

Studies have shown seniors that have chosen a healthcare center for themselves, either prior to a need or during, have a much better transition emotionally, a lower anxiety rate, and an extended life expectancy of an additional 3-5 years.

Some seniors have the means and desire to stay at home with private duty caregivers or a relative, but with the decline in the market recently, many seniors that had this as their main plan, suddenly may need to make adjustments.

Touring these centers can assist the hospital or rehabilitation center staff, and/or your primary care physician in making sure your choices are honored in the event they are needed. Many healthcare living centers offer parties and lunches at no charge to help introduce their community to the public.

For instance, some whom are living in their home and declining, may have family arrive from out of town on a visit, who suddenly realize how care they actually now require, and begin the process of choosing a center for them, usually in panic mode, and much against their will.

Resulting in a much more difficult transition, given the personalities involved, than if a senior is able to chose for themselves an Independent, Assisted Living or Skilled Nursing Center.

With so many different types of healthcare settings available, let's examine the variety of options with the objective to search more efficiently.

There are often local counties that have different senior living magazines and websites featuring many of these communities that are available, and usually at no charge.

Many seniors believe that the only choice they have is home or a "nursing home", however, there are so many more options for senior living than ever in our nation's history.

INDEPENDENT LIVING CENTERS & SENIOR APARTMENT LIVING

These communities require that their residents be able to perform most of the activities of daily living independently and without assistance.

Activities of daily living are eating, bathing, dressing, toileting, transferring (walking) and continence.

These very basic mandatory requirements are crucial to a senior being able to live safely in these communities. Some residents also still own and drive a car in senior apartment living and independent communities. Most are also "pet friendly" as long as the pet is a certain size and up to date with vaccinations.

The monthly rent usually includes meals, housekeeping, local transportation and social activities. Most independent living centers also have some nursing services or a home health agency available if medications need to be managed. Senior apartment staff may offer connections to outside resources when more care is needed.

Most of these centers try to attract very healthy and active seniors without the need for a cane or walker to get around. Choosing this type of community early is recommended as this can help maintain a senior's independence and activity level.

Independent Living Centers or Senior Apartments offer very minimal assistance.

Most of these communities charge rent monthly, with an annual contract. The charges will vary based on location, and the amenities offered. The benefits to the residents are that they usually have access to transportation, housekeeping and social activities.

Also, there are many Continuing Care Retirement communities that offer the same services, some on a month to month rental basis, and others with a "buy in" option.

There are also low income properties that offer this style of living and only charge a percentage of the senior's social security income, and /or assets, which can be a great option, especially if the only income is social security or a small pension.

ASSISTED LIVING CENTERS

These centers provide much more assistance with the activities of daily living than Independent living centers or senior apartment communities. They do require that the resident be able to transfer with supervision only, depending on the type of license they have, and the licensing requirements of the state they are located in.

In some states, there are advanced assisted living licenses that allow them to perform more assistance, such as a "limited nursing" or "extended congregate care" licenses. These licenses allow them to manage diabetes, and provide more assistance with a resident's activities of daily living.

Many Assisted living centers also offer day care usually costing around $50 – $150.00 per day which is a nice way for a senior to get familiar with their services and community.

Some also offer short term respite stays, which is another way of exposing a senior to the center without actually having to move in.

The cost for assisted living centers vary based on the area and the amenities they offer.

Many are pet friendly, and will allow a dog or cat to be less than 25 to 35 pounds. Of course, they usually require that the resident be able to care for their pet, however, some places offer pet care at a nominal charge.

Some states offer assistance paying for assisted living care under their Medicaid program. We'll cover the Medicaid coverage in a later chapter.

Shopping for Assisted Living is much like shopping for a car, do so late in the month, if possible and feel free to negotiate the monthly rate. Also, it's helpful to make the rate good for a year to be sure that there are no unexpected rent hikes later.

<u>Alzheimer's Assisted Living Centers</u> are assisted living centers that are secured and have activity programs to assist residents with the symptoms of Alzheimer's disease or dementia. The requirements for these centers are usually the same as assisted living with the key difference that the residents usually are at risk of elopement requiring a secured environment for their safety.

There are 7 stages of Alzheimer's with dementia as the condition that usually identifies this diagnosis.

These centers are considerable more expensive than most Assisted Living Centers, however, depending on the area, some do accept state Medicaid programs, if allotted by the state budget for care.

The local Alzheimer's Association chapter offer support groups that can assist in referring the caregiver and family to local facilities that offer this type of assisted living, either on a short or permanent basis.

The website below can help you to find a local chapter.

www.alzfdn.org Alzheimer's Association

www.alfa.org Assisted Living Federation of America

www.caring.com/assisted-living

CONTINUING CARE RETIREMENT COMMUNITIES (CCRC)

This is a community that offers all levels of care, Independent, Assisted Living and Skilled Nursing and Rehabilitation center. They are either a monthly private pay fee or a buy in community, and in some cases, a combination of both.

The advantage some find in these communities is that a resident can transition to the next care level as their healthcare needs increase.

The warning for a "buy in" communities are that some seniors have bought into them, at a substantial fee, and have not been pleased with the services, or found that they never needed the amount of care levels they had paid for.

Most Independent and Assisted Living centers are on a month to month rental basis, especially due to the uncertain nature of a seniors future health needs. The freedom and flexibility of a monthly rent system can be appealing to many seniors as they have the ability to change their surroundings if they become unpleased with the care or require more help.

WE'VE CHOSEN A CENTER, HOW DO I GET MY LOVED ONE TO AGREE TO MOVE IN?

To start, many seniors that need more care than they can have or afford at home refuse to accept any changes in their environment. Some seniors are in denial of their care needs, forcing the adult child to become the parent. You wouldn't allow a child to determine their care needs and although it's very difficult to do, an unreasonable senior, especially with any kind of safety issues, should not be making these decisions either.

One way to get a senior to try a long term care center is to go on vacation, and have them stay at a center on a short term / respite basis. It sounds selfish, but this is one way to allow them to try an active retirement center without forcing an actual move. Most places offer a respite package, and this can be either a weekend or longer. Many times when a senior is moving into a long term care setting, their house may need repair. I've recommended tenting the house, renovating bathrooms or kitchens if needed to motivate them to stay at a preferred center, on a trial basis.

Most seniors comment after moving into a center they now realize that they should have done this a long time prior, and have reported they feel more energetic than before. The tough love approach, while not easy, is still in their best interests.

SKILLED NURSING & REHAB CENTERS aka "NURSING HOMES"

Skilled Nursing and Rehab Centers provide both short term rehabilitation, and long term custodial care. The short term rehabilitation includes physical, occupational, speech therapies, IV medications and wound care and much more. The long term residents living in skilled nursing centers are usually residents that need assistance with most if not all of their activities of daily living.

Most seniors that need short term rehab in a center do go back to their home, or an independent or assisted living facility, depending on the care needs of the patient upon discharge.

Not all Skilled Nursing & Rehab centers are created equal, and it's important to tour and see the condition of the residents living there to make informed choices in advance.

The most urgent decision that causes a lot of stress on families is when a loved one is at the hospital, and they're told that the doctors want their loved one to go to a Skilled Nursing & Rehab center. Sometimes they've been discharged and they need a decision NOW, or YESTERDAY. They will sometimes decide for the patient if a facility has not already been chosen.

Therefore, knowing in advance a place that is preferred, takes the urgent stress out of this type of situation.

Every state has an inspecting agency and a website that can help find out what the most recent survey results were, as well as any penalties or fines. It's still best to tour personally as a lot of the information online can be quite out of date.

http://www.medicare.gov/nursinghomecompare

When touring a skilled nursing center, the touring form listed next can be most helpful.

TOURING "Nursing Homes"

What type of deficiencies did the center receive at their last state inspection?

_____

How often is physical therapy provided?

_____

What is the percentage of residents that are long term versus short term rehab?

_____

What insurances does the center have contracts with? _____

Does my physician have rounding privileges here? _____

What is the staff to patient ratio (<u>some states regulate this</u>)? _____

How many patients discharge home weekly?

_____

What are the biggest complaints the residents in house have? _____

_____

(Make copies for multiple facility tours)

Aside from the "sniff test", note how the residents are dressed, and their overall appearance. Observe the staff, how attentive they are to the current resident's and their overall happiness with their job.

If possible, talk to some of the current residents and ask them about their day.

No matter how good a rating a center can have by the state rating agency, it only takes a change in management for that status to change, despite the ratings.

For instance, there was a 5 star rated facility that was put on a national focus list meaning they were being surveyed by state and federal inspections every 6 months due to their lack of compliance. So although they had in the past been a 5 star rated facility, that status had dropped drastically, yet the website (3 years old) continued listing them as a 5 star facility.

If your instincts are telling you that this isn't a good fit for you or your loved one, trust your instincts. Most staff would prefer not to admit someone against their wishes, as usually the transition is much more difficult for all concerned.

HOW DO I MOVE A LOVED ONE OUT OF A CENTER IF A DIFFERENT ONE IS PREFERRED?

So, let's say that the research has been done, and you or your loved one, want to move to a different center. How do you get them moved?

First, all of these centers with the exception of senior apartments and Independent living centers require a written physician's order of some kind. The form a physician has to fill out are state specific, however, the admissions department of every Assisted Living and Skilled Nursing and Rehab centers will know and have these forms.

The process usually starts with the center you prefer making a determination that your loved one has and/or, will be accepted. To allow the new center to do an evaluation simply let the Administrator or Social Service Director know that another center will be coming in to evaluate. Most centers will not accept a new resident sight unseen, unless they are coming from out of the area.

Once the new center has the required paperwork, transportation simply needs to be arranged. Most centers do NOT cover the cost of transportation, and neither Medicare nor Medicaid will pay for a "center to center" transfer. If you or your loved one requires an ambulance, that can become quite costly. It's important to evaluate the care required, and count the cost.

Sometimes, attempting to reconcile with the current center can change you or your loved one's experience.

If you encounter any resistance from the current center regarding making a transfer or in resolving current care issues, you can also call in your local Ombudsman officer to try to mediate. Ombudsman is part of the National Long-Term Care Resource Center.

It's key to remember that some seniors are not going to be happy anywhere they are, sadly. If the care has suddenly changed for the worse, it's also good to find out if a new corporation has purchased them.

Most Assisted Living and Skilled Nursing Centers are owned by a handful of the same corporations. Moving your loved one from one healthcare center to a different one that is owned by the same company may not increase your loved one's experience.

Many of the reasons why care can change in an Assisted Living or Skilled Nursing and Rehab Center is directly linked to what they pay their nursing staff. If a new corporation has taken over that pays less than the current market rate, it can create a great degree of turnover, which also can result in the declining care.

Most importantly, it's important for families and extended families to have a strong presence in whatever center their loved one lives in to ensure the highest and best care.

202-332-2275   National Long Term Care
                  Resource Center / Local
                  Ombudsman

FACILITY LIVING SUMMARY

The more prepared for additional health care center needs, the better. Handling these choices before they're needed can make a senior's experience drastically better and even more so when they're involved in the decision making.

In some areas, there are companies that offer to serve as a liaison to assist families in making a choice in senior housing options. They usually offer this service at no charge to a senior or family, but may charge the facility a fee, such as one month's rent, depending on the state laws.

At times, if there are multiple family members that can't decide, these liaisons can serve as an unbiased voice to outline the pros and cons for each place.

To summarize, the best defense is a healthy defense!

AGING IN AMERICA

WHAT YOU *NEED TO KNOW* ABOUT NAVIGATING OUR HEALTHCARE SYSTEM

Chapter 3

ESTABLISH ADVANCE DIRECTIVES WITH A SUPPORT TEAM *BEFORE NEEDED*

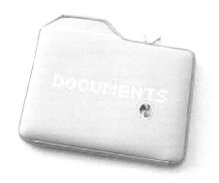

* Living Will * Do Not Resuscitate (DNR) * Healthcare Proxy

* Durable Power of Attorney (DPOA) *

WHAT ARE ADVANCED DIRECTIVES AND WHY ARE ESTABLISHING THEM SO IMPORTANT?

Advance Directives are your specific healthcare wishes put into writing in the event that you become unable to express your wishes for yourself. It explains to your loved ones and medical professionals exactly what medical measures you want taken, or NOT taken, in the case of an unexpected medical emergency or medical condition that causes you to be unable to speak for yourself.

Many believe that because they know what or how they would like to be medically treated, if the need arises, that those people closest to them will know as well.

How many times, perhaps watching a movie or witnessing a real life experience, we may think "I would scream if they put me through that"? Probably as often as we hear the evening news, or watch a medical show on television.

That's why having Advance Directives spelled out in writing is so very important. If your loved ones don't have your wishes in writing, they can't make sure that you are taken care of the way you would like.

Many have mistakenly thought that "my loved one knows what I would or would not want DONE to me," only to find out later that there are huge misunderstandings.

This situation happened to me personally. There was a very public medical case that drew nationwide attention that let me know that my healthcare proxy did not agree with my personal wishes, put in the same situation.

This very sad case had the media reporting the dispute in that the parents wanted their daughter to have a feeding tube in her stomach (peg tube), and her husband fighting against it.

This tragic and heartbreaking case brought to light that my own personal Healthcare proxy (my mother) needed to be changed.

It's a good idea after writing out Advance Directives to make sure they are discussed and understood by all involved. It's very important to make sure all clearly understand what certain medical phrases mean.

Many seniors have suffered in ways they did not want, simply because they never reduced their wishes in writing in a clear and easily understood way.

LIVING WILL

A living will is very different than a financial Will, which outlines the distribution of financial assets in the event of a death.

A Living Will outlines very specifically what conditions a person wants taken to preserve or not preserve their life. This is vital in communicating to the medical community HOW and WHAT medical procedures are preferred to in a medical emergency. The forms are listed at the websites below, and may be state specific.

This document makes a person really decide about what types of medical treatments they would want taken, one way or the other, and most importantly, makes it so that you or your loved one chooses, instead of the medical community, and helps medical professionals comply with personal wishes.

It's ok to add to a living will phrases like "no tubes", "hospice care welcome", "comfort measures only" for example.

The more specifics are on this document, the better.

DO NOT RESUSCITATE (DNR)

When a person is making decisions for their Living Will, most often the Do Not Resuscitate (DNR) becomes up for discussion.

This is a document that states that in the event of a non responding medical condition, the medical professionals are NOT to resuscitate the patient.

Until a patient is made a "Do Not Resuscitate" (DNR), they are a FULL CODE status, meaning the medical staff will use all available methods to resuscitate the patient. Thus, if a patient stops breathing, ALL methods will be used to save a life.

This may include having a tube down your throat or cracking open your chest to assist you in breathing.

This status at times creates confusion for many families. If someone has chosen to have a Do Not Resuscitate (DNR), it does NOT mean that the medical professionals no longer treat the patient medically. It simply means if they stop breathing, they will not be using EXTREME measures to resuscitate them. It does not mean 'DO NOT TREAT". There are still many treatment choices that will need to be made.

Such routine decisions can include treating infections, as simple as inserting a more permanent IV port, or as serious as deciding to have a more serious surgical procedure.

There are many hard decisions that have to be made at the end of a person's life and very careful and clear communication assists staff in making the best decision possible when these occasions arise.

This is why the person chosen to protect a person's healthcare choices is so important.

The person chosen to protect basic medical choices has to be the most reliable and ethical person possible.

The reason why that person is so important is covered in the later on in this book, and that is THE SECOND most important choice anyone can make.

HEALTH CARE PROXY vs. DURABLE POWER OF ATTORNEY (DPOA)

Regardless of what state you live in, these are the two most common legal forms of designating a person to decide important medical and financial matters for you in the event you can't speak for yourself.

These forms can be the most difficult to decide. Healthcare Proxy is a form that gives a person power to decide healthcare decisions for you, and only healthcare decisions for you, and ONLY in the event the patient cannot speak for themselves.

Durable Power of Attorney is a legal document that gives someone power to utilize bank accounts to pay bills, execute important business decisions, and make healthcare decisions, in the event they cannot perform such tasks personally.

For instance, there may be a family member or close friend that may be trusted with financial decisions but not healthcare decisions, and vice-versa.

It's ideal to have a trusted family member be able to be Healthcare proxy and Durable Power of Attorney (DPOA) however, this is not always available or wise.

Because this person holds power over finances, and healthcare needs, this person needs to be chosen very carefully.

I've seen perfectly legal yet horrific things happen to people by their legal Durable Power of Attorney.

DURABLE POWER OF ATTORNEY (DPOA)

This form was established to assist families to conduct financial business for a loved one who may not be able to take care of things during a medical emergency.

*This person should be the **MOST TRUSTED AND FINANCIALLY STABLE FAMILY MEMBER OR LIFETIME FRIEND**.*

The enormous amount of power this person has, involving both healthcare and financial decisions, means that they need to be a very trustworthy person.

Some have abused this power to their own financial benefit, and at times to a senior's detriment.

Having a family member that is struggling financially is not a great choice for this role, as the temptation to take advantage may result in a senior not being taken care of.

It is very possible to have one trusted family member as the healthcare proxy, and another different family member as the Durable Power of Attorney. These forms on occasion may need to be changed, and should always be given to the person that's chosen for their records.

These forms should be easy to find, in the event of an unexpected medical emergency. These forms will also need to be given to any medical professionals in the event of an emergency.

BELOW ARE SOME SAMPLE WEBSITES FOR EACH STATE SPECIFIC FORM:

www.caringinfo.org

www.aarp.org

www.putitinwriting.org

www.edmedicinehealth.com

www.agingwithdignity.org

www.nlm.nih.gov/medlineplus/advanceddirectives.html

AGING IN AMERICA

WHAT YOU *NEED TO KNOW* ABOUT NAVIGATING OUR HEALTHCARE SYSTEM

CHAPTER 4

PUT ALL FINANCIAL & HEALTHCARE PREFERENCES IN WRITING

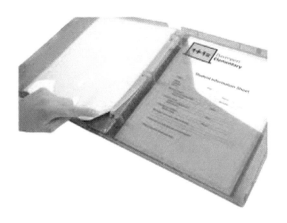

"Writing is of all arts, universally admitted to be that which is most useful to society. It is the picture of the past, the regulator of the future, and the messenger of thought."

IMPORTANT PAPERS IN SEPARATE BINDER / FILE (EASY TO FIND)

Now that we know the different Advanced Directives and paperwork that can be crucial to a senior having their wishes upheld, we need to get a practical system that a family will need to have access to.

Since seniors are living longer, and there are so many more choices than in previous years, it's very important that all wishes are put in writing.

Also, it is extremely helpful if they are easily accessible for the family or support system.

Ideally, it's best to have 3 ring binder with all of the most important documents readily available.

It should have all advanced directive documents, Healthcare Proxy, Durable Power of Attorney documents, a Do Not Resuscitate (if one is in place), as well as local banking contact information. If there is a family or Elder Law Attorney that has helped with these documents or financial affairs, their contact information should also be included.

If a financial will is in place, some seniors have their attorney hold on to it, or in a safety deposit box to avoid any family members fighting over belongings.

Many Husbands/ Fathers have always handled all the financial affairs, and unfortunately some wives have not had access to the specific finances. Subsequently, if the husband/father has a sudden medical condition that renders him unable to communicate these specifics, a 3 ring binder can help the family know how to conduct business on their behalf.

Many families have experienced many unnecessary bills because the family member that has become ill is unable to conduct business as usual, and no information has been shared with the family members.

Certain banks will not conduct business, even necessary business, with family members unless these legal documents are presented.

This suggestion may sound simplistic to families that have open communication and have an organized game plan in the event of an emergency. With so many families in the "sandwich situation" raising their own families and managing an aging parent, the time to get around to these very important papers can make life much simpler when they're needed. This can be very difficult if the aging parent is private about financial matters.

For families with estranged relationships that haven't been mended, the result can be even more severe for a senior.

When should these matters be setup for a senior? The answer comes down to their general health. There are healthy, active seniors that live to 90 plus years; however, they are the rarest of our population. If a senior has had multiple medical conditions at a young age or have experienced the following medical conditions: high blood pressure, high/low blood sugar, cardiac problems, obesity, arthritis, joint disease, kidney problems, cancer or any other major disease that requires medication, the time is <u>NOW</u>, or <u>YESTERDAY.</u>

Checklist for Binder

- ➢ **Living Will**
- ➢ **Do Not Resuscitate**
- ➢ **Healthcare Proxy**
- ➢ **Durable Power of Attorney**
- ➢ **Bank Account Information**
- ➢ **Life Insurance Policies**
- ➢ **Family or Elder Law Attorney contact information**
- ➢ **** Secure Financial Will ** (Attorney or Safe Deposit Box)**
- ➢ *Fact: Many Seniors are not aware that Medicare will pay for an ambulance trip.*

AGING IN AMERICA

WHAT YOU *NEED TO KNOW* ABOUT NAVIGATING OUR HEALTHCARE SYSTEM

CHAPTER 5

ORIGINAL MEDICARE vs. A MEDICARE ADVANTAGE PLAN:

HOW TO MAKE THE BEST CHOICE

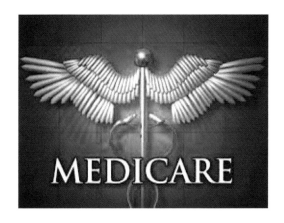

"You are free to choose, but you are not free from the consequences of your choice!"

ORIGINAL MEDICARE versus

A MEDICARE ADVANTAGE PLAN "HMO"

While writing this chapter and waiting for my car to be fixed, I overheard an adult child and her aging mother discussing weather she should get on Original Medicare or a Medicare Advantage Plan when she turned 65 next month. Of course, I stopped to help them understand what factors are essential in making this decision.

Many people do not realize that in America medicine is BIG BUSINESS, NOT A HUMAN SERVICE. Many times people fight the idea of socialized medicine; however, the countries that have successfully established it, consider healthcare a human service. In those countries doctors are paid by preventative care percentages, and their citizens, for the most part, do receive what they need without going broke. Obviously, not all countries have mastered the kinks out of their healthcare systems, but America does remain one of the few countries where one major illness or hospital stay can deplete a person's savings and/or result in bankruptcy. The same principle applies to receiving Medicare benefits when eligible.

Thus, the decision to have Original Medicare or a Medicare Advantage Plan is a BUSINESS ONE. There are essential factors that need to be carefully considered when making this decision. First, let's understand how Medicare works.

MEDICARE is a federal health insurance program for eligible individuals. It has no spousal / dependent coverage and does NOT cover long term custodial care. It's administered by the Centers for Medicare & Medicaid Services (CMS).

ELIGIBILITY REQUIREMENTS: You must be a United States Citizen or legal, permanent resident of the United States for at least 5 continuous years prior to enrollment. You must be at least 65 years old or if under 65: receiving Social Security disability income for at least 24 months, or have End State Renal Disease (ESRD) or Amyotrophic Lateral Sclerosis (ALS) "Lou Gehrig's Disease".

ENROLLMENT is coordinated by the Social Security Administration (SSA), or Railroad Retirement Board (RRB).

- Initial Enrollment Period: 7 months prior to 65th Birth month.
- General Enrollment Period: January 1st through March 31st. Coverage starts July 1st.
- Annual Election Period a.k.a. "Fall Open Enrollment": October 15th through December 7th. Changes effective January 1st. For those already in Medicare, join or switch Medicare Advantage Plans, return to Original Medicare, or add, drop of switch Medicare Prescription drug plans.
- Special Enrollment Periods: Original Medicare – working past age 65 with Employer Group, moving out of plan's coverage area, Involuntary loss of coverage, Qualify for Medicaid Assistance.
- Medicare Advantage Disenrollment Period:
- January 1st through February 14th. Disenroll from any Medicare Advantage Plan and return to Original Medicare with optional stand alone drug coverage.

WHAT ARE MY MEDICARE CHOICES?

There are two main ways to get Medicare Coverage: Original Medicare or a Medicare Advantage Plan.

Use these steps to help decide on a coverage plan:
Start

Step 1: Decide how you want to get your coverage.

Original Medicare   or   Medicare Advantage
                                                    Part C "HMO/PPO"

Part A – Hospital Insurance
Part B – Medical Insurance   Part A, B & usually D

Step 2: Decide if you need to add drug coverage.

Part D – Prescription Plan   Included in most
                                                    plans

Step 3: Add supplemental coverage?

           END

Medicare Supplemental   Can not buy a
(MEDIGAP POLICY)   Supplemental
                                              Insurance Policy

ORIGINAL MEDICARE: PARTS A & B
"Fee for Service"

➤ Can go to any provider that accepts Medicare (usually anywhere).
➤ No authorization required for any Inpatient or Outpatient Care.

❖ **Part A** – covers Inpatient Hospital Care, Blood, Skilled Nursing Care, Home Health Services, and Hospice Care. 80 – 100% medically necessary services covered.

❖ **Part B** – covers Doctors Services, Outpatient Medicare, Durable Medical Equipment, Preventative Services. 20% co-payment due on most services.

❖ Does not cover Vision, hearing, dental, travel coverage, private duty nursing, or long term custodial care.

ORIGINAL MEDICARE COSTS

Part A
➤ 2014 Premium: Free for most (need 40 work credits)
➤ 2014 Hospital Deductible $1216.00

Part B
➤ 2014 Premium Cost: $104.90
➤ 2014 Annual Deductible: $147.00

High Earners Part B Premiums
➤ Single Earners ($85000 - $107,000) $146.90
➤ Single Earners (over $214,000) $335.70

MEDICARE SUPPLEMENTAL/ "Medigap"

- ➢ **Pays for payment gaps in Original Medicare (co-pays etc.)**
- ➢ **Provided by Independent Health Insurance Companies (costs vary).**
- ➢ **All benefits have to be the exact same, regardless of differing costs (shop diligently)**
- ➢ **Enrollment Period: Up to 6 months following Medicare Part A & B.**

Cannot be denied due to health conditions.

MEDICARE ADVANTAGE PLANS "Managed Care"

- ➢ **Part A & B Services covered (co-payments may apply).**
- ➢ **May reimburse for part or all of Part B premiums.**
- ➢ **May include Prescription Drug Coverage.**
- ➢ **May include Vision, hearing, dental, travel etc.**

  - ❖ **Must use in network Primary Care Physician and providers.**
  - ❖ **May charge high daily Co-Payments for hospital, Skilled Nursing Centers, and some specialty treatments and surgeries.**
  - ❖ **Requires authorization by Insurance Case Manager or Primary Care Physician for specialty physicians.**
  - ❖ **Requires authorization for home health services.**
  - ❖ **1 year mandatory trial period. (May disenroll if relocating).**

Enrollment Period: October 15th –
December 7th
Disenrollment Period: January 1st –
February 14th

PRESCRIPTION DRUG COVERAGE (Part D)

This coverage is available to all Medicare recipients. Stand- alone Medicare Drug Plans (PDP) supplement Original Medicare. The Affordable Care Act will be closing the "donut hole" that required seniors to pay more for their medications until benefits began to pay. It's predicted in 2014 that those that qualify will receive a 47.5 percent discount on certain brand name drugs and a 21 percent discount on generic drugs until they reach the out of pocket limit.

Medicare Advantage Plans with Prescription Drug Coverage (MA-PD) offer a variety of plans that members can choose from based on their personal health needs. Some Advantage Plans support and serve the prescription drug benefit, and some require their members to purchase from independent insurance companies.

Under the Affordable Care Act, 2014, higher income Medicare beneficiaries (those who earn more than $85,000 per person or $170,000 per couple) will pay slightly more for their prescription drug coverage. This change is expected to affect about 5 percent of beneficiaries.

These costs need to be included in any Original Medicare or Medicare Advantage Plan chosen.

WHICH MEDICARE PLAN IS BEST?

Some seniors and families have found out the hard way that not all Advantage Plans are always "advantageous" for them. This decision can be very confusing to make, so let's make it as simple as possible.

The Insurance companies (the wealthiest industry in the world for a reason) are in the business of making and saving money. So they receive money from our government to provide services Medicare offers to their beneficiaries, at a profit. They also have extremely large marketing budgets, and sales tactics that can be very confusing to seniors and their families. First tip, the Insurance Company with the larger marketing budget is not necessarily going to be the Company that provides the most benefits.

Most states do offer a <u>DEPARTMENT OF ELDER AFFAIRS and possibly a SHINE program (Serving Health Insurance Needs of Elders).</u> These programs are available to help guide and counsel seniors having to make this decision, and can be an excellent tool in counting the cost to determine which plan is the most "advantageous" route to take.

Some Medicare Advantage plans reimburse some or all of the Medicare Part B premiums, and many seniors struggling to survive on social security and/or shrinking pensions are often tempted to save money by joining one. Furthermore, if a beneficiary is in good health, they may receive many offers from different companies. The company benefits when their members are in good health, as they lose money by having to authorize costly hospital and specialty treatments.

In a nutshell ~ MEDICARE ADVANTAGE PLANS ARE FOR HEALTHY PEOPLE. So if you're in reasonably good health (no hospital stays, serious diseases, chronic diseases, etc) they can be an affordable option, especially if there are no large assets or pensions to live on.

Seniors living strictly off of their social security income and/or social security disability income may qualify for their local state community Medicaid. One key change with the Affordable Care Act is that the local State Medicaid Program has been expanded, and many that may have been denied in the past, may now get approved.

Most State Medicaid programs pay what Original Medicare does not pay in co-payments, and prescription drug coverage. Many seniors meet the poverty requirements to be eligible for Medicaid in their state, however, have never applied.

APPLY, APPLY, & APPLY!

To be directed to your local state website:

www.medicaid.gov

(See Chapter 6 Understanding State Aid Programs)

CHOOSING A MEDICARE ADVANTAGE PLAN

First of all, if you decide to go with a Medicare Advantage Plan, you no longer have Original Medicare, as that option has been waived.

Members of a Medicare Advantage Plan are at the mercy of the Insurance Company they have chosen. They will assign a Primary Care Physician, and most authorizations will go through that office. Any tests, procedures, specialists, hospital, skilled nursing and home care will need to be authorized by them.

The primary care physician may have a "full risk contract" with the insurance company which means that the doctor receives a monthly amount per patient from the insurance company (usually $5 to $10 per patient), whether they see the patient or not.

In some cases, the doctor also receives more money if they don't authorize some costly tests, and/or specialty consults. Also, they usually have a Nurse Manager in the field that rounds on any of its members that are in any local hospitals and sometimes in their homes. This case manager will usually offer suggestions and decide what home care services or rehabilitation center therapies that a patient will receive.

So when weighing the cost of Original Medicare versus a Medicare Advantage Plan, weigh the costs very carefully. For a relatively healthy senior, this can be a good alternative to Medicare Part B premiums, however, understand that once there are hospital stays especially with any major illnesses, they will be looking for ways NOT to pay. This means there will be more out of pocket costs. On the first hospital stay or treatment for any serious medical condition, it's wise to disenroll from any Medicare Advantage Plan and return to Original Medicare.

The hidden costs to members that are in a Medicare Advantage Plan are usually discovered when a hospital stay, skilled nursing care, costly tests, therapy services or home care are needed.

For instance, a lot of seniors whom are in a Medicare Advantage Plan do not know that they will have a daily out of pocket co-payment at a Skilled Nursing and Rehab center, sometimes from day one, and will only be able to receive care at the Insurance Company's contracted centers (which may or may not be preferred).

If it's decided to go with a Medicare Advantage Plan, there are some quality companies. The locally owned companies tend to offer more consistent care benefits, however, may not be beneficial when traveling. Some local, not nationwide, Medicare Advantage Plans are owned by physicians, and may have the human compassion when authorizing needed medical services.

The large, nationwide Medicare Advantage Plans enjoy the largest marketing budget and the higher number of members, and have at times been the WORST at authorizing what their members require. How else could they afford the best marketing commercials, etc? They make better profits when their members are healthy, not sickly.

When dealing with a Medicare Advantage Plan, you do get what you pay for. The more the company offers in the beginning, the less they will pay for later.

Also, the nationwide Medicare Advantage Plans usually have lower reimbursements for their physicians and ancillary providers, who are the trying to save money to maximize their reimbursement by not authorizing or providing the necessary services.

These are the doctors that routinely ask what Insurance a patient has when they see them at an appointment. A quality physician should be treating all patients according to the standard practice of medicine, regardless of their insurance.

Let me give you some examples, a 65 year old patient who had a hip fracture and surgery, found at the hospital that their Medicare Advantage Plan's primary care physician was refusing to authorize physical therapy in a rehab center due to the fact that the patient smoked, and wanted to send her home with Hospice, and throw in the towel. The family appealed, and won.

Another Medicare Advantage Plan's Nurse Case Manager refused to authorize skilled nursing care in a center on a patient who had a stroke because he also had dementia, which is a very common condition for seniors.

These are just a few examples of how they save money later, and under Original Medicare Skilled Nursing and home care therapies that are medically necessary are approved without need for any authorizations. Usually under Original Medicare there are longer benefits that can be given, as long as the physician deems the patient requires it.

If a Medicare Advantage Plan is denying something that Original Medicare pays for, always appeal. If the primary care physician is in a "full risk contract" with the insurance company, they may be of little help. Legally they have to resolve an appeal within a specific number of days, given the circumstance, and the patient has the right to review their appeal decision. This process is not an easy one to win. That is why if it appears a senior will need intensive home care or rehabilitation services in the near future, Original Medicare is always the better option.

Many seniors think they will NEVER need any assistance in the future, near or far, and avoid any reminders to the contrary. It might be human nature and a desire to live forever. The reality is that most illnesses are not a sudden surprise. There are usually gradual clues that a person is declining. Any new medications prescribed for a serious medical disease is a sign of the possibility of needing more healthcare services in the future, and a good time to begin the disenrollment process from a Medicare Advantage Plan getting back on Original Medicare.

HOW DO I DISENROLL FROM A MEDICARE ADVANTAGE PLAN?

This can feel like quitting the post office, and can be very hard to accomplish.

The disenrollment period is from January 1st through February 14th annually. However, anyone is able to disenroll when they qualify for State

<u>Medicaid program, as well as if they're going into
a skilled nursing and rehab center.</u>

The customer service representatives are instructed
to keep as many members as possible, and may not
be very helpful. If possible, finding a kind hearted
person in the doctors office to help, as they usually
have an inside person they deal with daily. Also, it's
best to send multiple written requests to them by fax
and certified mail. They will always process a
disenrollment request easily once they think a
member needs long term skilled nursing care, as
they won't want to be having to authorize therapies,
medications, etc.

Many people think that Original Medicare is too
expensive, and may not realize that they are eligible
for state Medicaid programs, depending on their
monthly income, that may pay for Medicare Part B
premiums, co-payments, and medications.

Original Medicare is still the easiest, open network
with the most freedom to go to any physician,
hospital, home care and Skilled Nursing and Rehab
center.

Contrary to what may be said around election years,
<u>NO PHYSICIAN IS GOING TO REFUSE A
MEDICARE PATIENT.</u> It's still one of the highest
paying insurances in the country, with the least
hoops to jump through.

Original Medicare as a primary insurance, with a
supplement (if it can be afforded) or State Medicaid
as a secondary is the only and best way to be sure
there will not be costly deductibles and co-payments
due later.

Those inside the local healthcare community know that most physicians WILL NEVER REFUSE A MEDICARE PATIENT, regardless of whoever is the President of the United States!

In summary, count the cost carefully, and always try to get the most information from any Medicare Insurance professional that can help with the best prices.

For more information regarding Medicare Options:

800- MEDICARE   www.medicare.gov   Medicare Service Center

866-226-1819   www.cms.gov   Centers for Medicare & Medicaid 800-677-1116

www.eldercare.gov   National Agency on ELDERCARE 800-772-1213

www.ssa.gov   Social Security Administration 800-963-5337

800-96-ELDER   Department of Elder Affairs SHINE (Fl)

www.longtermcare.gov
US department of Health & Human Svc.

QUESTIONS TO ASK A MEDICARE INSURANCE AGENT

Can I continue with my primary care physician or will a primary care be assigned to me?

_____

What happens if I'm out of state and need healthcare? _____

What hospitals and skilled nursing centers are contracted locally, and out of the area? _____

_____

Are there any daily co-payments if rehabilitation services are needed after a hospital stay? If so, how much and on what day do they begin?

_____

Is there a "Tier Level" for authorizing Prescription drugs? _____

How much home care is usually authorized after a hospital stay? Is there only one company that is contracted, or will there be choices? _____

_____

What is the disenrollment process, should I wish to return to Original Medicare? _____

AGING IN AMERICA

WHAT YOU *NEED TO KNOW* ABOUT NAVIGATING OUR HEALTHCARE SYSTEM

CHAPTER 6

UNDERSTANDING STATE MEDICAID PROGRAMS: WHEN TO UTILIZE AN ELDER LAW ATTORNEY

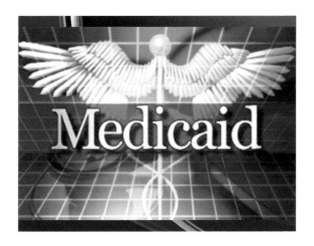

Medicaid is a "government insurance program for persons of all ages whose income and resources are insufficient to pay for health care."

(America's Health Insurance Plans (HIAA), pg. 232).

MEDICAID

"Enacted in 1965 through amendments to the Social Security Act, Medicaid is a health and long-term care coverage program that is jointly financed by states and the federal government. Each state establishes and administers its own Medicaid program and determines the type, amount, duration, and scope of services covered within broad federal guidelines. States must cover certain mandatory benefits and may choose to provide other optional benefits.

Federal law also requires states to cover certain mandatory eligibility groups, such as qualified parents, children, pregnant women with low income, older adults and disabled people with low income. States have the flexibility to cover other optional eligibility groups and set eligibility criteria within the federal standards. The Affordable Care Act of 2010 creates a new national Medicaid minimum eligibility level that covers most Americans with household income up to 133 percent of the federal poverty level. This new eligibility requirement is effective January 1, 2014, but states may choose to expand coverage before this date."
www.medicaid.gov

Every state has a Medicaid program that was implemented in 1965 by President Johnson. Each year, national and local government leaders make changes to this program to include more or less services offered. Each state has an online and in person application process for these services that can include healthcare, food stamps, medications, mental health treatments, and case management for low income families and seniors.

A person doesn't have to be destitute to qualify for some or all of the services provided, and can be a big help, especially if a senior is living on a low social security disability / incomes. Some seniors have regarded state aid programs with disdain, viewing it as a handout. However, these services are what their taxes have been paying into, for many years.

Seniors struggling to survive on small monthly incomes and/or shrinking pensions can benefit greatly from these state programs. Most seniors have been paying taxes their whole life, and are able to reap the benefits of being a law abiding citizen and get the financial help when needed.

Under the Medicaid Program there are different categories for seniors eligible for Medicare. They are listed below.

<u>Medicare Savings Program (MSPs)</u> is for low income Medicare beneficiaries and is coordinated in conjunction with any state Medicaid benefits. Medicare beneficiaries may qualify for their local state Medicaid in a variety of ways based on their gross monthly income and assets.

<u>Qualified Medicare Beneficiaries (QMB)</u> will pay Medicare premiums, co-payments, and deductibles at 100% for those with a gross monthly income of $958, and individual assets of $7080.00 or less.

<u>Specified Low Income Medicare Beneficiary (SLMB)</u> will pay the Medicare part B premium for those with a gross monthly income of $1149, and individual assets of $7080.00 or less.

Qualifying Individuals 1 (QI-1) will pay the Medicare Part B premium for those with a gross monthly income of $1293.00 and individual assets of $7080.00, or less. This division is very dependent upon the availability of funding.

Low Income Subsidy (LIS) is available for prescription drugs and for those that are blind or disabled. These benefits can be accessed through the Social Security Administration office, or www.ssa.gov.

All of these programs can be accessed either online at www.medicaid.gov or www.benefitscheckup.org.

Every state has different local agencies that can assist with the application process, and they may come by various different names. In Florida, the Department of Children & Families assist in the Medicaid application process, however, many seniors have dismissed their help, reasoning that they no longer have children at home.

Regardless of the state, Medicaid is a program to assist those living at or under the federal poverty level.

 Many states are implementing an initial online application, following with an appointment in person or over the phone. Any meetings in person with a state Medicaid office may require monthly bank statements proving any income and expenses.

Even if a senior receives too much in monthly income, and doesn't qualify for Medicaid, they may still qualify for food stamps or other services that can help ease the budget.

I met a widow struggling to make ends meet on a mere $800 a month social security, and had no idea how to pay for Medicare Part B premiums, and had not seen a physician in over 5 years. She had no idea that she qualified for her local state Medicaid. In her case, it was a decision of having to live with her family or remain independent in her apartment.

Each state has different requirements for the Medicaid program, however, many seniors that are struggling to survive, do qualify and have not known how to access these benefits.

Recently a family in Texas had their parents on a Medicare Advantage Plan, and their doctor would not authorize home care despite the desperate need for Dad, with an extreme care giving load falling on their Mother. They both qualified for Medicaid, after disenrolling from the Medicare Advantage Plan they were on thus returning to Original Medicare, the same doctor happily arranged for the home care help they needed. Original Medicare with Medicaid as a supplement offers the most freedom for care options, with the least money out of pocket.

In another case, a senior had many frequent hospital and skilled nursing / rehabilitation center stays. The Medicare Advantage Plan had been reducing the amount of benefits they would offer her, yet she was suspicious of disenrolling from the plan. Ultimately, she agreed, and was eligible for full Medicaid benefits, received her therapy and was able to return home with full assistance under Original Medicare, and no money out of pocket due.

Getting past a senior's feeling that Medicaid is a handout can be difficult, but many have benefited by these state programs for years.

The very worst that can happen is that the application for Medicaid is denied.

In short ~ APPLY, APPLY, and APPLY!

To be connected to your state's Medicaid website:

www.medicaid.gov

ELDER LAW ATTORNEYS

Elder Law Attorneys offer a wealth of different assistance for families that want extra life care planning, especially if there are assets that will need to provide for a spouse for years to come.

They can assist with all estate planning, probate, tax questions, disability, long term care, legal documents, advance directives, healthcare surrogates, financial wills, trusts, Medicaid planning programs, case management, and guardianships.

Most elder law attorneys charge approximately $2,000 - $20,000 or more given the size of the income and assets involved. Many states do allow for trust accounts to be established by family members so that a senior can qualify for Medicaid without depleting the family assets, especially if it may affect a spouse.

In some states, there are Medicaid Specialists that offer to help with setting up a trust and / or applying a loved one for Medicaid while preserving one's assets, especially if they are going long term into a Skilled Nursing Center.

If the income and assets are quite substantial, hiring an Elder Law Attorney is the wisest choice to protect those assets. They are experts at making sure all documents are current and accurate in accordance with the state laws.

Some families struggle when the assets have been depleted to under $100,000 and there may or may not be property involved. If an application to

Nursing Home Medicaid may be coming, it's still wise to hire an Elder law attorney. Some have tried to hire a Medicaid Specialist in these cases and they've had to pay the state restitution and fines. Especially if there is property of some value, it's better to hire an attorney.

If a senior is going long term into a skilled nursing center, and has relatively low assets and no property, using a Medicaid Specialist can be a more cost effective alternative, as they have considerably lower rates than an attorney. However, choose carefully as many Medicaid Specialist companies are highly unregulated, and may not have the expertise they claim.

Be very careful researching Medicaid Specialists, as in most states, there's little or no licensure required, and many have claimed they could get the people approved on Medicaid, to no avail.

Board Certified Elder Law Attorneys are preferred, as they've received additional training and have a license to protect. Word of mouth, online research and checking with the State Law Board can ensure that you're getting a reputable attorney.

To find an Elder Law Attorney in your area check below:

National Academy of Elder Law Attorneys 703-942-5711 or www.naela.org

AGING IN AMERICA

WHAT YOU *NEED TO KNOW* ABOUT NAVIGATING
OUR HEALTHCARE SYSTEM

CHAPTER 7

HOW TO ACCESS VETERAN BENEFITS

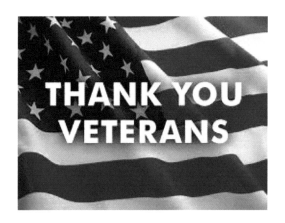

"It takes the courage and strength of a
warrior to ask for help"

VETERAN BENEFITS

Our veterans, regardless of age, many times are not aware of what benefits they are entitled to because of their service.

It has been astonishing to learn that for the men and women, who have sacrificed their life and safety for us, are not always aware that they have access to free to low cost co-payment healthcare at any local VA hospital, depending on their service connection status, and income criteria. Many get out of the military, and are never "debriefed" if you will, and some do not know benefits they are entitled to for life.

Some seniors have access to free or low cost healthcare at a local VA Hospital and never utilize it, either because they don't know they have this benefit or because they think they will receive substandard healthcare.

Most of the VA Hospitals are staffed with excellent medical professionals and are equipped with the latest medical tests, equipment and programs. However, some regions have better programs than others. Some VA hospitals offer a variety of specialty programs that are very unique and impressive.

Aside from having a primary care physician for care, veterans also receive free to low cost co-payments for any testing and medications they may need. They also can receive assistance for any mental health issues, such as Post Traumatic Stress Disorder (PTSD). For some veterans and their families, this is an extreme help to them financially.

The additional medical services veterans are eligible for are nursing, therapy, and social services in the home, oxygen, and medical equipment. The veteran has either free to low cost co-payments for these services depending on their service connection status and/or income criteria.

To get started at a local VA health care system it begins with enrollment. Veterans can now apply and submit their application for enrollment (VA Form 1010EZ) online at www.1010ez.med.va.gov/sec/vha/1010ez.

Veterans can also enroll by calling 1-877-222-VETS (8387) Monday through Friday,   8 a.m. to 8 p.m. Eastern Time, or at any VA health care system or VA regional benefits office. Once enrolled, they can receive health at any VA health care facility nationwide.

Veterans will need their DD 214, and have been honorably discharged to receive access to the VA healthcare system.

Each VA system has a Care Management team (OEF/OIF/OND) to coordinate patient care activities and ensure that Veterans are receiving patient centered, specific access to care and benefits they're entitled to.

While many veterans may qualify for free healthcare services, most veterans need to submit an annual financial assessment, to determine if they qualify for free services. A veteran whose income exceeds the established limits, as well as those who choose NOT to submit a financial assessment, will have to pay required co payments to be eligible for VA healthcare benefits. These co payment costs per physician visit and medications are very nominal.

Certain services are not charged a co payment at all. These apply to any publicly announced VA health fair or outpatient visits dedicated fore preventative screening such as vaccinations for influenza (flu) or specific diagnostic screenings, such as hypertension, hepatitis C, tobacco, alcohol, certain cancers, and HIV.

For some, a VA health care system may not be very close or easy to access. There is a reimbursement of travel costs that some veterans and/or their support system that they may be eligible for. In some cases, the VA will provide the needed transport (e.g. wheelchair van, ambulance when needed. Any transport eligibility can be coordinated through the Care Management team to determine if a veteran and/or their families are eligible for this service, and if any reimbursement travel costs are due.

Veterans and their families needing assistance to a wide range of information and services can also visit www.maketheconnection.net to find a place where stories can be exchanged, as well as information to connect to much needed assistance and veteran programs.

READJUSTMENT COUNSELING SERVICES

The VA offers readjustment counseling services through 300 community based Vet Centers nationwide. These counselors offer individual, group and family readjustment counseling to assist with the transition back to civilian life, however, also offer treatment for post-traumatic stress disorder (PTST), as well many psycho-social services including homelessness, medical referrals, employment, VA benefits, and the coordination of non VA services.

Any Veteran that served during World War II, the Korean War, the Vietnam War (some territory exclusions), the Gulf War, and some of the occupations during a combat time period, are eligible for these services.

Vet Center Combat Call Center (1-877-WAR-VETS) is an around the clock confidential call center where combat Veterans and their families can talk about their experiences, and any challenges they're having in adjusting to civilian life.

<u>MENTAL HEALTH CARE TREATMENTS</u>

There are many programs that provide support for Veterans dealing with a variety of mental health illnesses. The programs range from primary care clinics, home based primary care services to general and specialty mental health outpatient and inpatient treatment health units.

There are specialty programs for those with intensive mental health diagnosis that include a specific case manager, social worker, nurse and psychiatrist. In addition, the veteran may be able to access rehabilitation and recovery centers, work programs and homelessness assistance.

We've seen a growing number of aging veterans that may be struggling without knowing they are entitled to these programs, as well as their support system to help manage behaviors and increase in health care needs at home.

Veterans that need access to trained mental health professionals, need to call the Veteran Crisis Lifeline 1-800-273-TALK (8255). This hotline is available 24 hours a day, seven days a week.

Those in crisis may text 83-8255 free of charge to receive confidential, personal and immediate support.

www.mentalhealth.va.gov VA Mental Health Benefits

AID AND ATTENDANCE BENEFIT

This program is one of the best kept secrets in America!

Aid and attendance provides qualified veterans and their surviving spouse an additional income in ADDITION to any pensions they receive to pay for any home care or assisted living care they may require.

The program is based on many different government criteria, such as the following: the veteran must have served during a war, not an occupation (Vietnam doesn't count), need assistance in their activities of daily living either in the home or an Assisted Living Facility, written proof from a physician to that effect, and meet the service connection level that is required.

This money is in ADDITION to the Veteran's service or disability pension, and any social security or disability money the veteran is receiving. The additional pay (up to $1400 monthly) can be instrumental in affording the cost of medical care either in the home or at an assisted living center.

Each state has local Veteran Benefits Officers that assist at no charge in applying for this benefit at no charge.

There are also some companies that assist seniors and families in applying for this program at a fee. Any Elder Law Attorney would also be able to determine eligibility and help with the application process.

The veteran cannot receive this benefit if they require a Skilled Nursing and Rehab center.

Below is from the VA.gov website defining this program that senior veterans may qualify for.

"Aid and Attendance is a benefit paid in addition to monthly veteran pension and disability compensation. A&A can help cover the cost of in—home care, assisted living, or a nursing home.

This benefit may not be paid without eligibility to pension. A veteran may be eligible for A&A when:

- The veteran requires the aid of another person in order to perform personal functions required in everyday living, such as bathing, feeding, dressing, attending to the wants of nature, adjusting prosthetic devices, or protecting himself/herself from the hazards of his/her daily environment, OR,

- The veteran is bedridden, in that his/her disability or disabilities requires that he/she remain in bed apart from any prescribed course of convalescence or treatment, OR,
- The veteran is a patient in a nursing home due to mental or physical incapacity, OR,
- The veteran is blind, or so nearly blind as to have corrected visual acuity of 5/200 or less, in both eyes or, concentric contraction of the visual field to 5 degrees or less.

HOUSEBOUND BENEFITS

Like A&A, Housebound benefits may not be paid without eligibility to pension. A veteran may be eligible for Housebound benefits when:

- The veteran has a single permanent disability evaluated as 100-percent disabling AND, due to such disability, he/she is permanently and substantially confined to his/her immediate premises, OR,
- The veteran has a single permanent disability evaluated as 100-percent disabling AND, another disability, or disabilities, evaluated as 60 percent or more disabling.

A veteran cannot receive both Aid and Attendance and Housebound benefits at the same time.

Applying for Aid and Attendance and Housebound:

- You may apply for Aid and Attendance or Housebound benefits by writing to the VA regional office having jurisdiction of the claim. That would be the office where you filed a claim for pension benefits. If the regional office of jurisdiction is not known, you may file the request with any VA regional office.

- You should include copies of any evidence, preferably a report from an attending physician validating the need for Aid and Attendance or Housebound type care.
- The report should be in sufficient detail to determine whether there is disease or injury producing physical or mental impairment, loss of coordination, or conditions affecting the ability to dress and undress, to feed oneself, to attend to sanitary needs, and to keep oneself ordinarily clean and presentable.
- In addition, it is necessary to determine whether the claimant is confined to the home or immediate premises.
- Whether the claim is for Aid and Attendance or Housebound, the report should indicate how well the individual gets around, where the individual goes, and what he or she is able to do during a typical day." www.military.com/benefits/veteran-benefits/aid-attendance-and-house-bound-benefits.html?comp=1199433946637&rank=26

VA HOSPITAL & MEDICARE

Even if a senior has full access to a local VA hospital, they may still need to be on Medicare part B for to cover physicians and procedures that may NOT be available at their local VA Medical System.

Many seniors qualify for community Medicaid, which can offset any medical expenses should they need them traveling or for any procedure the local VA Medical System cannot provide for the veteran.

The American Legion locally also host fund raisers for veterans that need assistance, or are struggling financially. The local legions can be a great resource to additional programs the veteran qualifies for, as well as an excellent place to save money on food and drink.

The chief reason to apply for benefits is because the government uses the total number of veterans approved for benefits as a baseline for allocating money for the health care programs. Even if a veteran decides NOT to use the local VA healthcare system, it can still reserve a spot for a veteran in need in the future.

In short~ APPLY, APPLY & APPLY!

The links below can be utilized to see all veteran benefits:

http://benefits.va.gov/BENEFITS/factsheets.asp
                    Veteran Benefits Info

www.va.gov   VA Home Page

www.military.com   Military Branch Access
Website

www.nacvso.org/index.php   National Assoc. of County Veteran Service Officers

www.vba.va.gov   Veterans Benefits Association

1-866-260-3274   www.caregiver.va.gov   Caregiver Support

855-260-3274 Veterans Affairs – National Caregiver Support Line

800-273-TALK Veterans Crisis Help Line

AGING IN AMERICA

WHAT YOU *NEED TO KNOW* ABOUT NAVIGATING
OUR HEALTHCARE SYSTEM

CHAPTER 8

UTILIZING LOCAL CHARITIES &
NATIONAL HEALTH ORGANIZATIONS

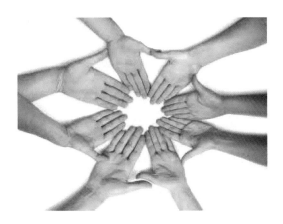

*"The Universal brotherhood of man is our
most precious possession." Mark Twain*

LOCAL CHARITIES

Every state and even every county within each state have different local civic and charity organizations. Some of these charity programs may be funded by the local governments, churches, or rely on local fund raisers.

These assistance programs may provide meals in the homes, nursing care, and transportation services to those that are homebound or are not able to drive.

Some of the states have had to make major cuts in their budgets and are cutting these charity programs that were extremely helpful in assisting those without health insurance.

Many disease based organizations that offer support group meetings will share information regarding local resources, free respite care, and even free medical screenings and services.

A lot of the local hospitals and senior centers advertise some of these programs when they are funded and available. However, some of these programs are only known to a select few working in hospitals. It's wise to attend some of the community educational lunches and programs that local hospitals offer for many reasons. For one thing, you may learn something new that will only benefit your overall health.

Secondly, establishing a personal relationship with a patient advocate or social worker that may have knowledge about resources can also prove beneficial for a variety of situations.

Knowledge is power, and the more that is known about choices and resources, the better.

The best way to find out about these local charity organizations is to search the internet with the key disease names or network with others locally. Also, social media can be very helpful as well.

Most hospitals have a facebook page, and if you "like" their page, you will be notified about upcoming seminars, screenings, and lunches. When you see an organization doing fund raisers at the mall, or other places, ask to be added to their email or mailing list.

If you or a loved one has a specific disease, make sure to register on their website and/or facebook page to be "in the know" on any upcoming events.

Some organizations provide meals, money, or free assistance to those that meet certain criteria financially or medically.

<u>NATIONAL ORGANIZATIONS</u>

The websites listed below are some of the national organizations that help people with certain diseases or conditions. For instance, some offer family members caregiver assistance; connect them with the local support groups and even money.

The Internet can be utilized to search any diagnosis that has been given, and receive information on local support groups and organizations that may have helpful programs.

When you or a loved one attends the support group meetings, you'll be in contact with people that have connections locally and nationally about all of the different programs these organizations offer. Since many of them receive federal funding, they can assist more people on a national level.

Years ago, the local Alzheimer's Association chapter provided free respite stays in an assisted living center for an Alzheimer patient, for a week or weekend. They would pay the centers directly. They also offered adult day care at no charge for families that needed a break from taking care of their loved one.

Once a person has been diagnosed with a serious disease, it's good to search out any national organizations that meet in the local area, and find out what resources they might be able to offer.

Below are some of the National organizations that can offer support and education:

800-772-3900   www.alz.org
        Alzheimer's Association

800- 227-2345   www.cancer.org
        American Cancer Society

888.322.8209   www.epilepsyfoundation.org
        Epilepsy Foundation

800-223-27323   www.parkinsons.org
        Parkinson's Foundation

800-342-2383   www.diabetes.org
        American Diabetes Assoc.

(202) 872-0888 <u>www.n4a.org</u> **National Assoc. of Area Agencies on Aging**

800-222-2225 <u>www.nia.nih.gov</u>
National Institute on Aging

800-677-1116 <u>www.ncoa.org</u>
National Council on Aging

AGING IN AMERICA

WHAT YOU *NEED TO KNOW* ABOUT NAVIGATING
OUR HEALTHCARE SYSTEM

CHAPTER 9

ACCESSING MENTAL HEALTH HELP

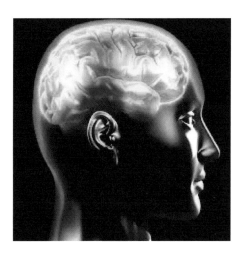

*"Healthy Citizens are the Greatest Asset
Any Country can have." Winston Churchhill*

It's ideal when any mental health issues can be managed on an outpatient basis. However, this is not always easy to do without first having an Inpatient hospitalization.

INPATIENT HOSPITALIZATION

For some families it actually takes an inpatient hospitalization to identify fully the cause for any changes in behaviors, or mental health diagnosis.

An inpatient hospital stay can help identify and treat any underlying emotional or medical reasons why the patient is declining. Because some psychiatric hospitals offer separated age and sex units, it can give a senior suffering with depression or other illness the chance to see that they are not alone in managing their emotions.

Due to the improvement in psychiatric hospital programs and units, some agree voluntarily to go for treatment.

The other arrival scene for inpatient hospitalization is when a patient is "Baker Acted" otherwise known as a BA-52.

What is a Baker Act?

Under the Baker Act law, any law enforcement officer, physician, clinical psychologist, psychiatric nurse, or clinical social worker, can take someone against their will to a psychiatric facility for a mental health evaluation if the person is a danger to themselves or others.

A person can't be held involuntarily for longer than 72 hours, and a medical expert needs to examine the person and sign off on his or her release.

It's notable that the simple act of being held under the Baker Act doesn't mean the person is mentally ill or in need of commitment.

In 2010, less than 1 percent of about 140,000 involuntary examinations led to involuntary placement in a mental health treatment facility, according to the Florida Department of Children and Families. This number doesn't account for people who voluntarily remained in facilities.

Under the Baker Act, people who haven't committed crimes are not supposed to be treated as criminals and they do retain their constitutional rights.

In many cases the 72 hour evaluations by physicians and psychiatric professionals can help identify any medication management, or other social service needs.

An inpatient hospital stay can also afford the family caregivers a respite, and identify if a change in environment is required.

CHANGES IN BEHAVIORS

A change in behavior can be a symbol of many things, both medically and emotionally. Simply because a senior may act differently does not necessarily mean they are suffering from a mental illness or any kind of dementia.

For many seniors a change in behavior or dementia like symptoms can be a sign of a urinary tract infection, dehydration, or other medical condition that requires medical treatment at a hospital.

In a situation like that, after antibiotic treatment the person's mental faculties may return to normal.

Since depression in this country is increasing in our senior population, it's vital that a primary care physician be notified if and when there are any sudden changes in behavior or personal losses.

It's also important to have any NEW medications scrutinized and make sure that they are not creating a change in behavior, or an unpleasant side affect. Especially when there are multiple physicians treating the senior, as one Dr. may be prescribing medications that are not cohesive to what they are already taking.

<u>It's crucially important at every physician visit that a complete and up to date medication list is included.</u>

Some families keep multiple medication listings so that if a senior is taken to the hospital suddenly, the medical professionals know exactly what they are taking.

CARING FOR AGING RELATIVES

The "sandwich generation" or those caring for their own families, while also caring for an aging relative are carrying a heavy load.

The guilt many adult children feel as a parent ages, needs more care, while denying that they do, can create confusing emotions. Some have confessed to having a "death wish" for an aging parent, and feeling guilty for having those feelings.

Many families struggle with the "when factor". When is the best time to talk with them about the care they need and who will take over financially.

Ideally it's best to work out these conditions early, before there is a need, and have a specific plan in place to honor the senior's wishes.

There are many caregiver relief organizations that can offer resources locally, as well as support groups to help support a family member while caring for an aging relative.

Below are some of the websites that can offer information and local resources:

www.aagponline.org American Association for Geriatric Psychiatry (AAGP)

www.alzheimers.org Alzheimer's Disease (ADER) Education & Referral Center

www.nami.org National Alliance on Mental Health (NAMI)

www.nmha.org Mental Health America

www.longtermcare.gov US Department of Health & Human Service

www.mentalhealth.gov HHS/Mental Health

www.samhsa.gov Substance Abuse & Mental Health Services Administration

AGING IN AMERICA

WHAT YOU *NEED TO KNOW* ABOUT NAVIGATING
OUR HEALTHCARE SYSTEM

CHAPTER 10

HOW TO PREVENT NEGLECT OR EXPLOITATION

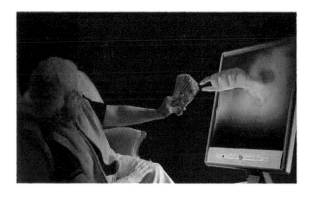

"Innocence is thought charming because it offers delightful possibilities for exploitation."

Mason Cooley, American Aphorist 1927 - 2002

WAYS TO PROTECT A SENIOR FROM NEGLECT & EXPLOITATION

According to the National Center on Elder Abuse, Bureau of Justice, there were over 5 million reported cases of abuse in 2010. That means that 9.5% of the senior population reported some sort of neglect or abuse in that year. There is no way to know how many UNREPORTED cases occurred.

Of the reported cases of elder abuse 58.5% were for neglect, followed by 12.3% for financial exploitation.

Interestingly, 67.3% were females with the average age being 77.9 years old.

Fast facts:

- ➢ The average exploitation per reported case is $128,288.
- ➢ For those with mental illness, that amount climbs to $143,068. If Medicare costs are included, that amount climbs to $171,600.
- ➢ The closer the exploiter is to the senior, the greater the average amount will be exploited.
- ➢ The average loss per case when an adult child is the perpetrator is $157,326.
- ➢ The average loss per case when a family member is the exploiter is $125,193 (a 47 percent increase more than the average exploitation).
- ➢ The average loss per case when a grandchild is the perpetrator is $45,496.
- ➢ The average loss per case when a paid caregiver is the perpetrator is $18,350.

➢ The average loss per case when the perpetrator has some sort of addiction issues (alcohol, gambling) was $25,688.

➢ The average loss per case when a stranger is the perpetrator is $30,219.

Methods of exploitation include both finances and property

Finances

➢ Scams
➢ Withdrawals from bank account(s)
➢ Cash
➢ Check (forgery)
➢ Credit Card (open debit card without knowledge, identity theft, or "borrowing credit or debit cards")
➢ Loans

Property

➢ Personal property
➢ House (stolen through transferring the property)
➢ Car theft or "borrowing"
➢ Rent (living off senior despite agreement)
➢ Medicaid (exploited senior now forced to be dependent on Medicaid

To prevent any financial exploitation, many banks offer seniors a third party oversight on any "shared" accounts, requiring the bank's approval on purchases. Many elder law attorneys also help in a third party role to oversee any real estate, or asset transfers. Having a trained and trusted professional as a third party overseeing any financial decisions is the best way to guard against exploitation, regardless of how trusted a Durable Power of Attorney may be.

Too many seniors in our country are taken advantage of by people they know and trust. These can range from neighbors, church groups, television shopping shows, and most of the time, their own family members.

How does this happen? It's a gradual process.

Most seniors try to maintain their independence for as long as they can, many times much longer than is safe to do so. They may have family members or a support system that will NOT take advantage of them financially, yet many do.

Some seniors have a family member that has recently lost a job, or are going through financial difficulties and see caring for an aging relative as a meal ticket.

This section truly breaks my heart.

On a weekly and daily basis we would witness sons, daughters, neighbors that can't afford to live on their own, move in with an aging relative to "help them out", only to later take advantage of them financially. Many times a senior may need more care than the caregiver can offer, and may block help that is desperately needed.

Many state aid long term care programs, such as Medicaid in a Nursing Home or Assisted Living Facility, have a requirement that to qualify for the benefit, the state will pay all healthcare costs for the senior, however, any monthly income they receive must be turned over to the center.

When an adult child lives with an aging relative, some have forgotten how to live within their own financial means. The dependence on that senior's income and/or assets develops over many years and can become quite difficult to sever when the senior's medical needs change. When this transition has to happen, they may panic, and in MANY CASES insist they can take care of their aging relative although they are physically not able to.

This is usually evidenced by repeat trips to local hospitals, and physician visits.

Since most seniors insist that they will leave their home "feet first" if you will, relatives can tap into that desire, and actually jeopardize their health needs rather than lose the additional income they've now become used to living on.

Seniors with mental illnesses are especially at risk. Recently, a very confused and homeless senior was baker acted into a hospital, and then sent to a skilled nursing center for physical therapy. All she had as an emergency contact was a "friend" / former neighbor of hers. We promptly proceeded to set up a Professional Guardian for her, however, not before we caught him trying to apply for a credit card with her social security number. These situations happen every day, sadly.

For those that may be shaking their head, or thinking, that will never happen to me, or my loved one, consider this. Many have been affected by our uncertain economy, and in some cases, when an adult child loses their job, and may be in a desperate state, will insist they can take care of Mom or Dad, to get their monthly social security or pension, even if they are not able to meet their medical care needs.

One case, a daughter of a nursing home resident lost her job, and although her mother had been living in the nursing center for many years insisted that she could take care of her mother at home. The nursing staff that had been caring for her mother for years was alarmed, and her physician adamantly objected, however, the daughter insisted she could take care of Mom at home. I asked the daughter, "You do realize that if she dies, you will not be able to live off of her income any longer, right?" She, of course thought I was being dramatic. Her mother was dead within 4 weeks.

To witness a senior go through their final moments not receiving the care they need is horrific.

In one case the son of a 92 year old woman learned how to "work the system" efficiently. As the woman was declining at home with her son, he would bring Mom to a hospital, subsequently get some rehab for her at a nursing center under her Medicare (100 days) and still keep her monthly income. He would also get a break from caring for her. He would bring her home on the 101st day, and start the whole process over with a different hospital in another area. However, as her condition worsened, he became increasing desperate, and ultimately the state authorities had to get involved to remove his involvement in her care.

One remarkable 78 year old woman, who was very hard of hearing, had been living with her daughter for many years at the time. However, as Mom's care became more demanding, the daughter was getting more and more afraid, insisting that she not lose her mother's $1400 monthly income. She had developed a system though. She would put Mom in 2 diapers in the morning when she went to work, leave her some snacks to eat during the day, and when she returned home 8-10 hours later, put her in another 2 diapers to last her the night. Obviously she developed wounds and when the state authorities got involved, this very deaf woman wrote on a piece of paper "I don't want to live with my daughter!"

Many families don't live near their aging relatives, and as the senior needs more help in the home, may hire a person locally to assist. They may be recommended by someone they know and trust.

One such example was what an adult daughter referred to me as "Helga the Housekeeper." The daughter lived out the area and her mother hired "Helga the Housekeeper" for shopping and cleaning needs. She gradually began to get more involved in her mother's life. She went as far as to take her to the bank to add her name to Mom's bank accounts, and had been stealing family heirlooms that she claimed were "given to her". In this particular case, the bank notified the family of the attempted change, and financial exploitation was avoided.

HIRING HOME CARE HELP

Many have made the mistake of hiring local help in the home only to find that the person has taken full advantage of their aging relative.

It costs more per hour to use a licensed private duty home care company, however, the staff they hire are usually bonded and insured, and had a positive background check.

Be very leery of private duty companies that have unfavorable state surveys, and/or multiple fines assessed. Since the more reputable companies do insist on clean background check to work for them, the chance is better that their staff will be more professional.

There are opportunistic individuals that intrude into senior living communities and offer help to seniors, and especially if they think family is not living nearby. Being proactive when an aging relative is needing help in the home will avoid them being prey to those that simply need a place to stay, or are in desperate need for money.

Statistics show that seniors living in Assisted Living centers live 3-5 years longer. This is due to the nutrition, socialization and nursing assistance. Therefore, when a caregiver for a senior is not open to this living alternative when they obviously require it, especially if it's being recommended by a physician, can also be a sign of some sort of possible financial exploitation.

This outlines the importance of trusting medical and financial decisions to the most responsible persons in a support system. They need to be financially independent themselves. Many seniors involve an attorney and / or bank officer as a third party to monitor both their finances and healthcare choices, just to be better protected.

The temptation by some individuals that have fallen on hard times to simply keep mom or dad at home when they are unable to take care of them, to have more income can appeal to those in a difficult spot financially.

Some cultures do not believe in a relative being taken care of by anyone except the family and I've personally witnessed families taking shifts to make sure their aging relative is taken good care of. These families are to be commended for their sacrifice, and great compassion.

Unfortunately, the opposite is what is being reported more and more. Since an elderly person can change so much as they reach their golden years, and can become much like a child, needing a tremendous amount of help, it's so important for families to have a REALISTIC AGING PLAN.

The families without a REALISTIC AGING PLAN are suddenly bounced around our healthcare maze, searching for answers and struggling to know where to go and what to do next. Hospitals have strict guidelines on how long someone can stay there, based on the insurance company involved, and will sometimes give families less than a day to decide on a rehab center, assisted living or home care support choices.

This is when the chaos and stress levels hit the highest levels.

What if you suspect that a senior is being neglected or exploited? Here are few signs that could mean they are vulnerable at this time or in some kind of a neglectful living situation.

- ➢ **Frequent hospital stays**
- ➢ **Social Isolation**
- ➢ **Bereavement**
- ➢ **Become very suspicious**
- ➢ **Changes in ability to perform activities of daily living**
- ➢ **Has an overly protective caregiver**
- ➢ **Seems fearful or distressed**
- ➢ **Financially responsible for Adult Child or Spouse**
- ➢ **Depression or mental illness**

Most states mandate that if you see or suspect neglect or abuse of the elderly to report it to the authorities at once. The take the alert anonymously, so the investigators make sure to protect the one reporting it.

If you suspect abuse of any human being, please contact <u>ADULT PROTECTIVE SERVICES   1-800-252-5400 (www.apsnetwork.org)</u> or your local police department which can then connect you to the correct organization.

Below are some of the websites that offer additional ways to protect an elder from neglect and / or exploitation.

www.ncea.aoa.gov   National Center on Elder Abuse

www.aoa.gov 800-677-1117 Administration for Community Living

www.211.org   United Way

www.seniors.gov 800-333-4636 USA.gov

www.cmsa.org/800-216-2672 Case Mgmt. Society of America

www.caremanager.org National Association of Professional Geriatric Mgrs.

www.caregiver.org 800-445-8106 Family Caregiver Alliance

www.longtermcare.gov   US Department of Health & Human Services

PROFESSIONAL GUARDIANS

A family suspicious of neglect or abuse for an aging relative, can also petition a judge to appoint a professional guardian. These are mediators that help protect those that need it, and have to report their findings to the court. They can also be useful to mediate a situation if differing family members can't decide on the right care for their relative.

Professional Guardians are sometimes called in when a senior has been the victim of neglect or exploitation. These are individuals that are ordered by a judge to care and make decisions for their "ward". Many times there has been family neglect or exploitation, or both, when they get assigned the case by the local authorities.

These individuals take a state mandated class to assist people that need some sort of assistance, either in healthcare choices or financial matters, or both. The difference is that all actions performed on behalf of one of their "wards" trusted in their care must be reported to a judge on a quarterly basis. They also are usually bonded and insured by the state, as most states do require this.

For some families that are disputing over the decision making of an aging parent (usually a wealthy aging parent) having a professional guardian involved can be a good alternative to family bickering. All parties would still receive an accounting of any funds used in the care of their relative and all involved can still visit and be involved however, there would at least be one neutral individual, the Professional Guardian, to make the final decision in question.

Most states and counties have an Elder Affairs department that can assist in contacting local Professional Guardians working in your area. Elder Law Attorneys work very closely with Professional Guardians and can be a great resource to find them.

www.guardianship.org   National Guardianship Organization

www.naela.com   National Academy of Elder Law Attorneys (NAELA)

SUMMARY

Fact: "Those who fail to plan can plan to fail."

Aging in America can be a daunting challenge and learning how to navigate our healthcare system is tricky. The main message here is to research and plan ahead.

Having the "talk" with an aging loved one may be uncomfortable but will save grief, money and reactionary behaviors later.

Many seniors that are declining may stubbornly deny that they need help when they do, and it's up to caregivers to make sure not to allow the health and safety of their loved one to be in jeopardy.

Making sure they are safe and prepared can assist the healthcare professionals greatly in providing the best of care when our seniors need it.

Understanding our healthcare system in our country can be an ever changing adventure, and the goal of this book is to provide as much information as possible.

Biography

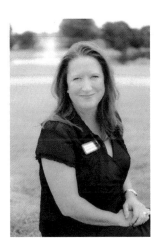

Karyn Rizzo, owner and founder of ELITE Marketing & Consulting has over 20 years in the healthcare industry.

A native of Chicago, Illinois, she has lived in Florida for over 20 years.

Her work in the Physician Office management and subsequently in the senior healthcare Assisted Living and Skilled Nursing Centers has created a unique outlook on the entirety of the industry. Her familiarity with all sides of the healthcare system, has given her a very unique perspective.

Her passion to help families connect to local resources and receive knowledge and assistance has been a key theme of her work over many years.

As a patient advocate in every sense, she has worked diligently to protect seniors and their families from those that would take advantage of them for their own personal gain.

This resource guide was meant to be an overall insight of our healthcare industry, and a very general overview of the key areas that may cause a real impact on an aging person's healthcare experience.

If you'd like to receive information and resources that are personal to your specific situation, send an E-mail message to the following website:

www.agingguidebook1.com.